DEDICATION

To Ken. Thank you for breaking my heart. When you did, I realized my strengths and now, I'm a stronger woman.

Table of Contents

Chapter 1- How to Lose Weight After Child Birth 5

Chapter 2- Breastfeeding and Losing Weight..........................11

Chapter 3- Is Post-Partum Exercise Safe?.........................15

Chapter 4- Eat Well, Not Less...............................20

Chapter 5- Quality over Quantity – Always..........................26

Chapter 6- The Principles of Weight Loss.........................32

Chapter 7- How Meal Timing Works........................38

Chapter 8- Getting Rid of a Mother's Nightmare – Belly Fat!......45

About The Author...52

How to Get Back Your Pre-Pregnancy Glory

Valuable Tips for Shedding Off the Baby Weight

By: Lisa Wright

9781635013030

PUBLISHERS NOTES

Disclaimer – Speedy Publishing LLC

This publication is intended to provide helpful and informative material. It is not intended to diagnose, treat, cure, or prevent any health problem or condition, nor is intended to replace the advice of a physician. No action should be taken solely on the contents of this book. Always consult your physician or qualified health-care professional on any matters regarding your health and before adopting any suggestions in this book or drawing inferences from it.

The author and publisher specifically disclaim all responsibility for any liability, loss or risk, personal or otherwise, which is incurred as a consequence, directly or indirectly, from the use or application of any contents of this book.

Any and all product names referenced within this book are the trademarks of their respective owners. None of these owners have sponsored, authorized, endorsed, or approved this book.

Always read all information provided by the manufacturers' product labels before using their products. The author and publisher are not responsible for claims made by manufacturers.

This book was originally printed before 2014. This is an adapted reprint by Speedy Publishing LLC with newly updated content designed to help readers with much more accurate and timely information and data.

Speedy Publishing LLC

40 E Main Street, Newark, Delaware, 19711

Contact Us: 1-888-248-4521

Website: http://www.speedypublishing.co

REPRINTED Paperback Edition: 9781635013030:

Manufactured in the United States of America

Chapter 1- How to Lose Weight After Child Birth

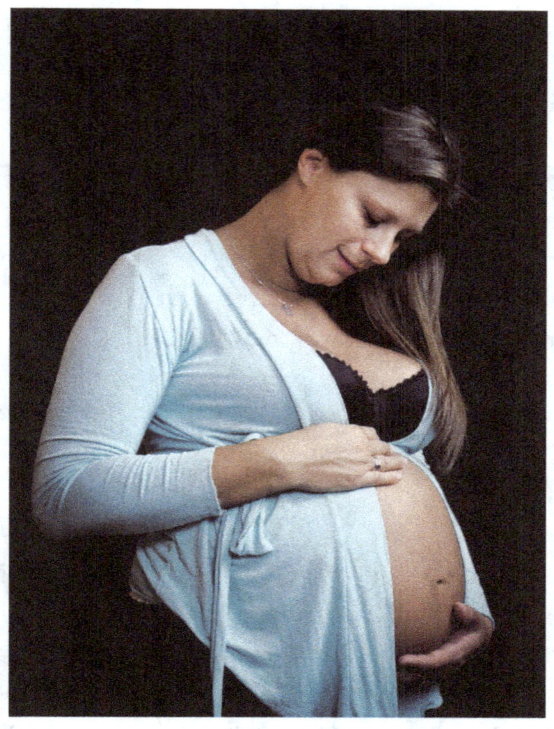

You've given birth to a new baby boy or girl; congratulations! There's no elation better. Likewise there's little disappointment greater than that of seeing your body in the mirror after returning home from the hospital.

On average, a woman gains between 25 and 35 pounds during her pregnancy. During and labor and immediately after delivery a new mother might shed 10 to 15 pounds of that. This leaves from 10 to 25 additional pounds of weight left on the new mom's "new" body. It can be a source of great shock, disappointment, frustration, and despair to a woman to discover that after giving birth she can no longer fit into the clothes she wore prior to the pregnancy.

How to Get Back Your Pre-Pregnancy Glory

Losing weight after pregnancy is not a fool's errand, but neither is it an easy errand; it requires patience, a realistic attitude, a positive outlook, and when it comes down to it – persistence and dedication. A realistic outlook by any means is to expect to lose no more than 1 or 2 pounds per week. For an extra 10 to 25 pounds, then, that can take anywhere from 2 months to 2 years.

There's no quick fix to losing weight after pregnancy – not a sustainable and lasting one, at least. So the best way to succeed is to start out with realistic expectations for the time frame in which to achieve your results and with the commitment to seeing the process through, however long it may take.

Now that you have the right mental attitude, let's go over a few suggestions for ways to get rid of that unwanted weight postpartum:

Don't start right away: Contrary to the "do it now" mentality you're normally advised to live by, when you've just given birth, your body needs time to adjust to the changes it's undergone over the preceding 9 months. Remember, you are not "returning" to the state you were in before your pregnancy; you're in a new state you've never been in before. You are in the body of a new mother, and this body needs time to get used to this new way of being. Avoid weight-loss dieting of any sort for a good three months after delivering. Don't worry about exercise so much as just being sure you remain active and moving around. You can use your menstrual cycle as an indicator of when your body is ready to take on a more intentional program of diet and exercise; when it normalizes, you're ready to go.

Start slow: Your body is still healing from the pregnancy, and diving headlong into a heavy-duty exercise regimen may be too much of a shock to your newly-adjusting system to do you any good at all.

Walking around the block or the park with your baby is an excellent way to begin, and it primes your body exquisitely for taking on more extensive and intensive exercise at a later date.

Set yourself up for success: That means keep your kitchen stocked with fresh and healthy foods, particularly snacks, so when you feel the urge to eat something, you have only suitable options around. Several smaller meals throughout the day will serve your ends far better than just 2 or 3 large meals. And don't try and starve yourself. You'll do no good to your new baby that way, and you'll invariably find yourself binging sometime later on to compensate.

Have patience with yourself. The period of time following pregnancy is already exhausting and exasperating enough, on so many levels. Don't burden yourself further with guilt, shame, and unrealistic expectations.

Shedding excess weight after pregnancy is not an easy task, but it can be done. Everybody is different. Rather than comparing your rate of postpartum weight loss to that of any other new mother, focus on sticking to the slow and steady path to the long-lasting results you crave: a body that glows more than it ever did during or before you got pregnant.

How Much Weight Did You Gain?

Weight loss following pregnancy and hanging up the tent sized maternity clothes is something all new mothers look forward to with anticipation. For most women, but for others, the baby fat is a bit more difficult to shed. Each woman is different and there is no "one size fits all" formula for shedding the weight gained during pregnancy. However there are a few weight loss guidelines to follow that will have the new Mom back feeling great and wearing her jeans once she gets her strength back.

How to Get Back Your Pre-Pregnancy Glory
How much weight did you gain during pregnancy?

The 25 pounds the average woman gains during a pregnancy are spread out more or less like this:

-Baby-8 pounds

-Placenta-1.5 pounds

-Amniotic fluid-2 pounds

-Breasts-2 pounds

-Uterus-2.5 pounds

-Fat, blood volume and water retention

If you were already a little overweight when you first became pregnant, remember that the numbers on your scale kept going to go up almost every time you stepped on it. Fasting or Weight-loss fasting diets following pregnancy are absolutely not a good idea.

How Do Celebrity Moms Do It?

What happened to that pre-pregnancy body you once had? After nine months of your body going through numerous changes, many of which you do not like or enjoy, your newborn is here and it's time to lose the excess weight you have most likely gained. You can speed the process of regaining your pre-pregnancy shape by exercising regularly.

While it may not help eliminate any stretch marks you may have, exercise will help you regain the body you had prior to becoming pregnant. Some of the most common questions asked by new moms are: How soon can one begin postpartum exercises? How long will it take to regain my pre-pregnancy shape? And what are the best exercises to help me achieve my goals? Keep in mind one of the most critical factors that help determine the answers to these questions is how healthy you were during your pregnancy - both physically and mentally.

Have you ever wondered how celebrity moms lose their baby weight so rapidly? One of the most common reasons is because they exercise strenuously prior to and during their pregnancy. Celebrities have been known to lose up to 60 pounds in what seemed like a few days. However, please keep in mind that this is not considered as the normal time frame. These individuals are also quite careful (almost to the point of obsession) about the types of foods they eat. They are also quite able to afford personal trainers and nannies so that they can perform their exercise routines 5-7 days a week for many hours at a time.

Because most new moms have the regular everyday tasks to contend with such as work, errands, families, losing that excess weight after childbirth is not quite so easy. Hopefully you found the time and the desire to engage in some kind of exercise during your pregnancy, even on the days you just wanted to simply crawl back in bed. If you did, you will find that the process of losing that extra baby weight will be a lot easier for you than for new moms who did no exercise at all while pregnant. Exercising regularly during your pregnancy will have given you the opportunity to become familiar with what will motivate you, give you the best results, and identify the types of exercise that you find the most enjoyable.

Walking, jogging, aerobics, yoga, and many other types of exercise will allow you to lose the extra weight more quickly and you will feel better at the end of each day. Having a new baby can be an exhausting task and the simple act of exercising regularly will undoubtedly increase your energy and stamina when you need it most. Most doctors will say that it is safe to start a post-pregnancy exercise routine six weeks after the birth of your child. Walking and swimming can be started shortly after your baby is born if you do so in moderate amounts at a slow pace. Work up slowly to the more strenuous exercises to ensure your safety and reduce the risks of any complications that could arise from over-exerting yourself before your body has had adequate time to recover.

Chapter 2- Breastfeeding and Losing Weight

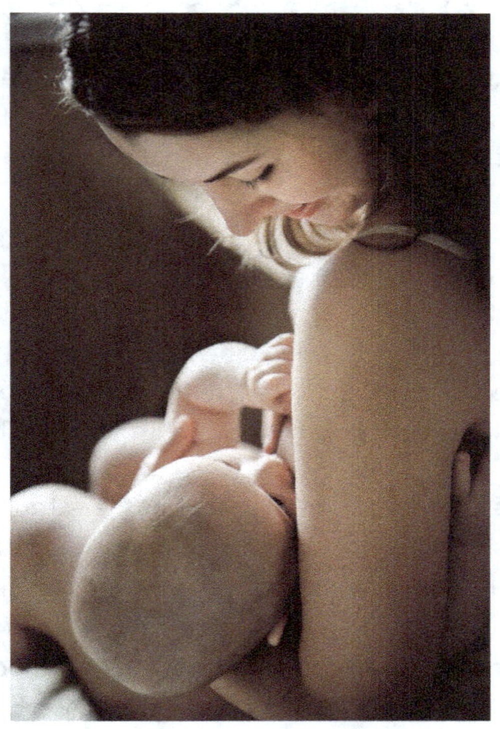

Many women who have recently given birth are always interested in attempting to lose some of that extra weight that traditionally accompanies having a baby. What many of these women do not entirely realize is the fact that breast-feeding can not only help provide the baby with essential vitamins and nutrients, but can also help in the weight-loss process. For example, the average mother will utilize somewhere between 500 calories and 800 calories a day producing milk for the baby. Not only will the baby receive the health and nutrition that it needs, but it may also enable a woman to lose baby fat a lot faster. As you can probably already imagine, it is a lot easier to say that going to the gym and cutting back on the amount of food that one need is the easiest path to losing weight.

That being said, it's not really a practical option for many new mothers.

There are a lot of responsibilities associated with having a baby which require a great deal of focus and effort. There's certainly nothing wrong with trying to eat healthy food and attempting to engage in some type of exercise on a regular basis. However, the point is that breast-feeding can really augment a new mother's effort to lose weight.

Remember, as mentioned a moment ago, between 500 calories in 800 calories a day are often consumed in the process of creating the milk that will be fed to the baby. Something that a lot of new mothers often times do is try to interact with other new mothers who find themselves dealing with a variety of similar challenges.

One of those challenges is losing some of the extra weight that is acquired as a result of the pregnancy. Women often times find it a lot easier to lose weight when they are able to communicate their peers and anxieties with other women and to support each other as they go about the process of shedding the extra pounds put on during pregnancy. In this regard, breast-feeding is a wonderful tool because he really doesn't require any extra effort. It's just something that naturally happens.

In addition to breastfeeding, taking walks and making an effort to eat low-fat food can really start to make a difference. As always, if in doubt, speak your doctor to make sure that you are doing what is best for your health as well as that of your new baby.

Cuarentea: A Latino Tradition after Childbirth

One of the best Latino traditions during the time right after childbirth is cuarentena, or the quarantine. The mother will spend forty days resting with the newborn after delivery and only worry about taking care of the baby. The new mother doesn't even consider weight loss issues during this time. Other members of the family will keep house and watch over the other children. While this may not be practical for most new mothers of today, if you do have relatives who live nearby, it would be a good idea to follow some version of this tradition. You'll feel like a new woman after those forty days of recuperation (or even twenty).

A nutritious diet is more important than weight loss for the first six weeks.

Pregnancy is a magical and mysterious time of life and many women worry about how to achieve weight loss after they give birth. During the first six weeks of postpartum, a healthy diet is much more important than a weight-loss diet. Continue to eat a balance of fruits, vegetables, whole grains, protein, calcium, and iron. Whether or not you're breastfeeding, your body is still recovering from the pregnancy and birth, and a nutritionally balanced diet will help you heal and feel better much faster.

Your care provider or doctor may recommend that you take an iron supplement for the first six weeks postpartum, while your body recovers. If you're breastfeeding, it's even more important to eat a well-balanced diet, since you're still sharing all the calories you're consuming. If you count calories, a breastfeeding woman should consume the same amount as she did before pregnancy to maintain her weight plus about 500 calories. For many, this means about 2,500 to 2,700 calories a day, which will support milk production and allow for moderate weight loss of half a pound per week.

Continue to avoid fish that are high in methyl mercury in your weight loss plan. Other foods, such as sushi, raw milk products, and deli meats, are less risky these days, but you should still take reasonable precautions to avoid food-borne illnesses. Precautions include cooking meat and poultry all the way through, washing all cooking utensils thoroughly, washing all fruits and vegetables thoroughly, and only eating raw foods like sushi from a dependable source.

CHAPTER 3- IS POST-PARTUM EXERCISE SAFE?

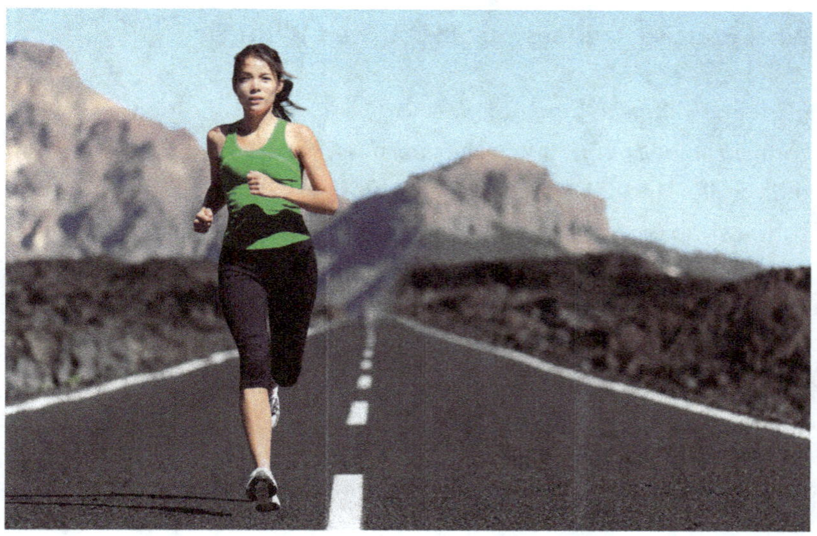

The six-week postpartum visit is a simple check-in with your caregiver or doctor. You'll be weighed, have your blood pressure taken, and you'll be asked about any problems. You will probably be given the green light on exercise.

Most caregivers recommend waiting until the six-week postpartum checkup before starting vigorous exercise, but that's a somewhat arbitrary time frame, based on the typical model of obstetric care. If you're stitches seem to be have healed, and if you want to be more active. Moderate exercise before the six week postpartum visit shouldn't be a problem

Listen to your body. Don't push yourself hard. Start out slowly, and if you find you're tired or uncomfortable, take your activity level down a notch. There is no reason to rush the healing process. There will always be time to exercise and address weight loss.

If you suffer from obesity, your doctor will tell you what kind of diet and exercise you should follow following the childbirth for weight loss.

What Exercise Routines Should You Start With?

It's a good idea to start taking short, easy walks as soon as it feels comfortable for you. If weather permits, simply load up the baby in the stroller and take brisk walks to the park, library, neighborhood coffee shop or anywhere that makes the exercise walk enjoyable. If you have a reliable baby sitter, joining a local gym would be an excellent idea.

The most important factors in weight loss after pregnancy will be patience and consistency, along with a sensible, healthy diet and an exercise plan. It generally takes about 6-12 months to achieve the total weight loss following pregnancy.

Yoga

I already see the raised eyebrows! However, did you know that doing hot yoga after pregnancy can not only help improve your psychological outlook, but can really have a lot of positive physical health benefits as well? Some of those positive health benefits that are physical in nature include burning fat and losing weight.

As you may or may not know, bikram yoga -- also known as hot yoga -- is a type of yoga that is typically engaged upon within a very hot environment. More fundamentally, when we talk about yoga we are talking about a series of movements that help the body develop internal calmness which can be really helpful for one's mental outlook while at the same time helping to expand one's strength and flexibility. When you combine these exercises with an incredibly warm environment -- typically around 95° -- you have a situation where a lot of calories can be burned in a relatively short amount of time.

That being said, it's also important to understand that you will need to focus on doing other things that will help you lose the baby fat Some of those other things include making sure that you are eating healthy food. Never try to starve yourself. Your body will detect this and become less likely to shed calories by actually going into stingy mode. You also want to make sure that you are doing reasonable amounts of cardiovascular exercise.

While it's certainly true that hot yoga will get your heart rate higher -- it is not really a substitute for taking frequent walks that will enable your heart to get some good exercise same time burning a lot of excess calories. Don't forget that you really need to work on your posture to improve your body image after pregnancy.

Bikram yoga is a phenomenal way to not only improve your posture and body image, but it will also really help you reduce the amount of anxiety and stress to you might be experiencing in your life. Although a joyful experience, giving birth to a baby can also create a lot of anxiety and stress. You owe it to yourself to spend some time focusing on your own health and wellness. If you have any questions about whether or not you are healthy enough to get involved with any type of yoga activity, be sure to speak your doctor. It only takes a moment, but it helps make sure that you're not doing anything that will harm you.

Relax: Take Some Time Out

Finally, far too many women want to try to lose the extra weight that they accumulated during their pregnancy virtually overnight. While it's certainly understandable that a woman would want to look the way she did before her pregnancy began sooner rather than later -- it's important that there be a realistic outlook on this process. After all, it takes approximately 9 months to gain the weight associated with being pregnant. Do you really think it makes sense to assume that most of the baby fat can be lost in nine days or less? Of course not!

Try to really relax and view this process as being something that will take at least two months. The reason why you want to try to view this as a long-term project stems largely from the fact that women who try to lose the weight quickly oftentimes find themselves feeling frustrated and upset by their apparent lack of progress. It's not even a question of them not making progress -- they usually are. But the progress is not fast enough to meet the unrealistic expectations that they have put on themselves. And let us not forget you are also doing this while caring for a newborn.

One of the easiest things that you can do is to set some very basic and realistic goals for yourself. If you do not establish goals, it will be far too easy to simply drift sideways and to assume that you're not really making any progress and to feel more anxious and frustrated about the entire process of losing weight after giving birth. Many medical experts indicate that losing approximately 2 pounds every seven days is reasonable for most women. When you do the math that works out to losing approximately 16 pounds in two months. While that may not be as much weight as you like to lose, you're giving yourself a realistic benchmark. If you happen to lose more weight than that, then that's great. It should mean that baby fat is melting away! But try not to stress yourself out over the process.

What many women fail to realize is that they can typically fall victim to something called emotional eating if they find themselves feeling stressed out an anxious over the weight-loss process. No woman wants to find herself in a situation whereby she feel so stressed out and anxious that she does the very thing which will sabotage your efforts -- eating excessive amounts of food. So as this process is approached, try to relax and realize that it's going to take some time to lose that baby fat.

CHAPTER 4- EAT WELL, NOT LESS

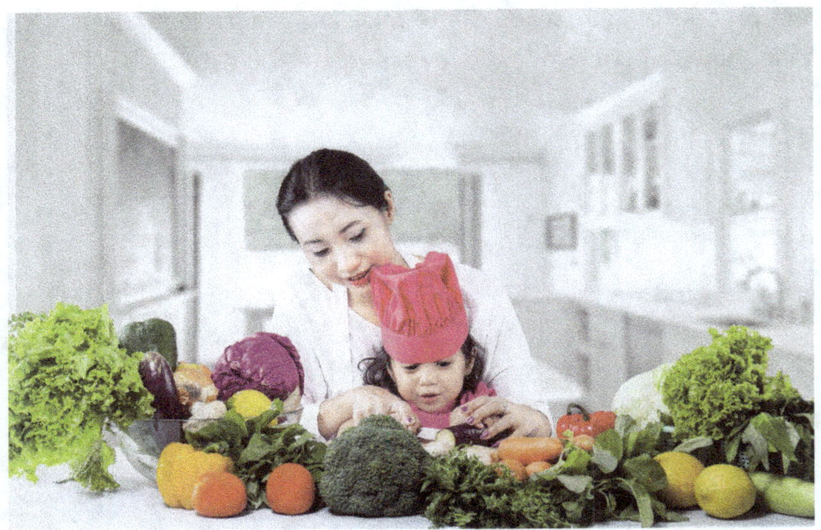

Next, many women who are interested in losing baby fat after giving birth will sometimes make the classic mistake of cutting back on the amount of food that they consume in a manner that is unhealthy. In other words, it can actually be counterproductive to eat dramatically less amounts of food if you are truly interested in losing weight. The reason why this can be so problematic is because your body will automatically detect that an unusually lower amount of calories are being consumed. This will typically result in a situation whereby your metabolism will slow down.

In essence, your body becomes far more efficient at being able to process the calories you do consume and restricts the amount of calories that are burned throughout the day. What this basically means for a new mother is that she will not experience the type of weight loss she is expecting. By cutting back too much on the amount of food that is being consumed, a woman who has just given birth can not only be potentially affecting the health of her baby -- assuming she is breast-feeding a baby -- but it is also causing a situation whereby her body will not shed as much weight as she thinks it will.

Other downsides associated with restricting the amount of calories you consume include feeling tired, cranky, and not really having the energy to do things. This also includes not really having sufficient amounts of energy to partake in reasonable amounts of exercise that all health experts agree to be very beneficial to losing weight. The real solution in a situation like this is to make sure that you are eating well. This is not to suggest that you should eat a bunch of junk food or otherwise mistreat yourself by consuming vast quantities of food that really have nothing to do with making sure that you are getting sufficient calories, vitamins, minerals. The idea here is to instead fill yourself with the calories you need but not an excessive amount of calories.

Finally, make sure that you engage in some type of exercise on a regular basis. This can be something as simple as taking walks. What few new mothers realize is that breast-feeding a baby can also help burn up to 800 calories per day. Eat well, do some exercise, and consider breast-feeding your baby. All these things will help you lose much of the extra weight that you accumulated after childbirth.

Drink Lots of Water

Drinking plenty of water is something else that can dramatically help a new mother lose weight. How is this possible? And to be realistic, how much weight can actually be lost using this method? Let's dig into this issue. The very first thing you need to understand is that water has no calories whatsoever. We are not talking about special water that you might buy at a grocery store that contains sugar or other additives which contain calories.

The water we are referring to is the basic water they can come right from the tap. You may be wondering why it is significant that water has no calories. When you stop and think about it, we all need to drink something. Why drink a beverage that contains calories if your goal is to lose baby fat? Most medical studies have strongly suggested that the overwhelming majority of people will get all the hydration that they need from water.

You don't need to drink sugary sodas to become hydrated. This raises the question of whether or not diet soda is a suitable alternative to water. After all, the amount of calories contained in diet soda can be extremely low. What you need to remember is that a lot of scientists have concluded that your body performs better and is less likely to develop problems related to excess weight when you drink water. In addition, there are a lot of artificial sweeteners that are used in various types of soft drinks. This could have a negative impact on your baby assuming that you are breast-feeding.

Drinking water is not enough. You need to also make sure that you have the type of lifestyle that will help you lose weight and keep it off. Considering the fact that you are a relatively new mother, it may not really be practical for you to be spending a lot of time at the gym or otherwise carefully following a very detailed diet. However, it really helps if you can do a little bit of exercise every day. This can have a dramatic impact on your ability to lose weight in conjunction with drinking plenty of water and eating reasonable portions.

In the final analysis, women who are interested in losing weight after giving birth to a baby need to take a multidimensional approach to solving the problem. This will include drinking plenty of water, getting some exercise, and eating well. Doing all these things will produce remarkable results.

Stop Eating for Two

When you were pregnant, you may have eaten more than usual to support your baby's growth and development. Proper nutrition is still important after the baby is born - especially if you're breast-feeding - but your needs and goals are different now. Making wise choices can promote healthy weight loss after pregnancy. Focus on fruits, vegetables and whole grains. These foods provide you with many important nutrients while helping you feel full longer. Other nutrient-rich choices include low-fat dairy products, such as skim milk, yogurt and low-fat cheeses. White meat poultry, most fish, beans, and lean cuts of beef and pork are good sources of protein, as well as zinc, iron and B vitamins. These foods will help in your weight loss program.

1. Avoid Temptation- Buy healthy foods at the grocery store and don't keep junk food in the house.

2. Eat smaller portions - Don't try starving yourself or skipping meals. Just cut back on the portions.

3. Eat only when you are hungry - Distract yourself with an activity if you are constantly hungry.

4. Drink water before meals.

What is the Calorie Deficit Approach?

Right now, if reports from health agencies are accurate, there could be a billion people in the planet experiencing weight problems. The health and fitness industry which generates billions of dollars in health related revenues continues to churn out various weight loss programs based on drastically reduced calorie diets along with strenuous workouts, and you wonder why the obesity rates are still increasing and whether such an approach is really effective.

Many of the makers of these programs, of course, stress that in order for them to work you heed to persevere, be disciplined and have the tenacity to persist in the face of difficulties that said programs are liable to bring in.

Perhaps the difficulties that you have to undergo when employing these weight loss routines is the main problem which means that all along makers may have been selling an approach that hardly works in the first place. Lose weight fast? You or anyone else for that matter will have a hard time resisting that kind of marketing pitch.

Fortunately, some weight loss advocates are trying to shift approaches, from low-calorie diets to less stressful methods. And they base the shift on something that's simple and logical – calorie deficit.

When you are overweight, it only means one thing; you have fat deposits in your body that your metabolism can't process. The question is why your metabolism can't do that. The answer is you are taking more calories than your metabolism can handle. Does this mean that you have to starve yourself in order to lose weight? Of course not, you will be risking your health if you do that and you will end up dealing with worse problems than before.

The key to losing weight without experiencing a whole range of issues is to create a calorie deficit, which simply means that you eat fewer calories than your body demands. Fewer calories are the keywords, not zero-calories. When you take in fewer calories and you work out, your body starts burning your fat deposits to supply you with the energy you need for the workouts. Naturally when your body burns fat deposits every day you will not be far away from your ideal weight.

Advantages

The calorie deficit approach has many advantages that are not present in drastically reduced weight loss diets. You do not need specially prepared meals to ensure the required calorie intake levels. All you need to is to eliminate some of the calorie loaded foods you are in the habit of eating. Your body won't be deprived of energy which allows it to function normally and you will feel good as you lose weight.

Aside from reducing the calories, your diet has to be as nutritionally balanced as you can make it. You want the natural body cleansers in it to help your metabolism work more efficiently. You need the proteins and other nutrients that promote good health.

Benefits

One of the benefits of the calorie deficit approach to losing weight is your health is never compromised; instead, you can become healthier. And unlike low calorie diets that make it difficult for you to protect gains because the deprivation will make the foods you used to eat hard to resist, with this approach since its slower the diet will be a habit by the time you have realized your weight reduction goals.

CHAPTER 5- QUALITY OVER QUANTITY – ALWAYS

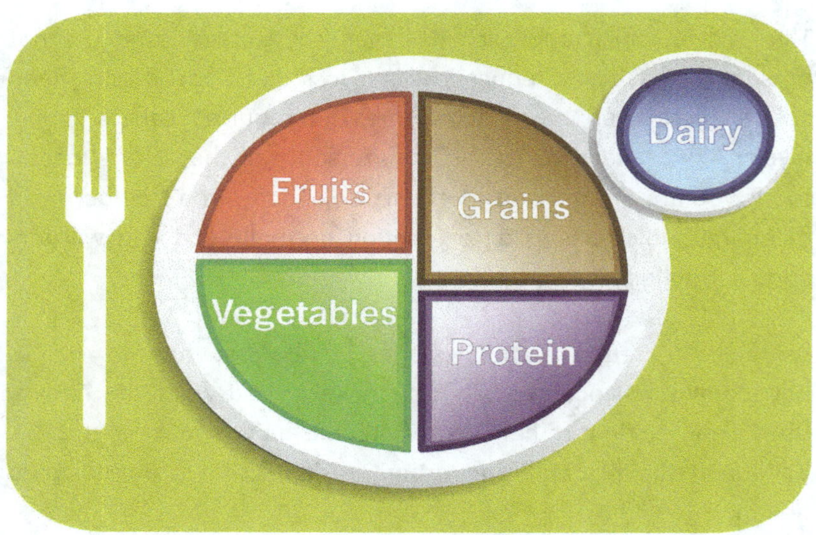

When trying to lose weight, dieters tend to focus on the quantity of the food they intake. If you are one of these people wanting to shed pounds, listen up. Here's something that you need to keep in mind:

CHOOSE QUALITY OVER QUANTITY ALL THE TIME.

Most people on a diet tend to drastically cut down on food. Some even starve themselves thinking if they do not eat food, they won't gain weight. Sure, that is true. However, it will also not help you lose weight. In fact, if you stop eating, your body will work on keeping your fats so that you can have the energy you need during the day.

So what does a person have to do? What is the right quantity of food to eat during a diet? How often can a person eat? All of these questions will be answered in this article, so continue reading on.

Most experts say that there are many more benefits when it comes to losing weight if you eat 5-6 meals per day compared to 3 meals. Granted the meals are small, of course. The reason for this is because your body will have balanced levels of sugar in the blood. Meaning, you won't be feeling intense hunger. When a person is hungry, they tend to eat more than usual.

Eating smaller portions throughout the day will also reduce cholesterol. In studies done by experts, it was proven that having smaller meals consumed 6 times a day decreased cholesterol levels by 5 percent.

Fill that Plate Up With the Right Kind of Stuff

What a person eats greatly affects their weight loss or weight gain. This is why dietitians encourage people to go for quality over quantity. A good example is you might have eaten only crackers for lunch today but also had a huge jug of sweetened drinks. Then that sweetened drink is the culprit when it comes to your weight gain.

If you had a large bowl of fresh salad and water, then that would have been considered a better meal on a diet than the crackers with a sweetened drink. It is much better for the body to take foods that are less in carbohydrates. Taking away bread, pasta, rice or potatoes and replacing it with vegetables will definitely help cut back on fat.

If you are the type of person who will feel full only if you see large portions of food on your plate, then the solution is to fill your plate with the right kind of food. Think colorful fruits and vegetables.

Deep colors means higher content of vitamins, minerals and antioxidants. All of these are what your body needs every day.

To commit to a long-term diet, it is important to like what you eat. If you hate the thought of just eating vegetables or fruits all day, then do some research on diet recipes. Eating meat is encouraged, so don't cut back on that. As long as it is not always deep fried, then it's still good.

It's really important to enjoy the process. Otherwise, you will easily go back to your old routine. Just remember, too much of anything is bad. Keep everything well balanced and eat only when your body is telling you it's hungry.

The Importance of a Balanced Diet

In a world where fast food is considered a real meal, no wonder there are so many people in a bad shape. The rate of obese people is a cause for alarm but this can all change if everyone gets educated on healthy eating habits.

The secret to healthy eating is all about balance. It's having all the right nutrients, vitamins and calories in one meal. There's really no need to deprive yourself from food that you like. It's about having all of these foods, but in moderation. Like the old saying goes: "Too much of anything is bad." This can be applied greatly to the food you eat.

The truth is, what you consume everyday greatly affects your whole attitude and energy level for the whole day. Sure it is convenient but there's so much more to life than a cheeseburger meal or Chinese food take out. It's tasty and you can't help craving it, but experimenting in your kitchen can easily result in the best meal of your life.

So here are some tips for healthy eating habits for a better you:

If you are just starting to change into a healthier lifestyle, then do it slowly. Your body has been accustomed to old ways and if you change drastically, it is likely that you will also give up easily.

Eat At Home

Whenever you eat out, you do not have any control on the portions that you will have. You might end up eating more than you need to.

Do Not Skip Meals

If your goal is to lose weight, then it is much better to eat small portions of food 5- 6 times a day. Skipping meals will only retain the fat in your body and may result in overeating.

Snack Healthy

When you're feeling hungry, instead of reaching out for the cupcake, grab that carrot stick instead. Some good examples of food to snack on are fruits, nuts, raisins, cranberries, whole grain crackers, etc.

Enjoy Your Meal

Do not rush the eating process. Take your time and chew your food slowly. When you're already feeling full, then stop eating. Listen to what your body tells you.

Along with these tips, you should always remember to have not just good eating habits but also a healthy lifestyle. This means making an effort to exercise regularly. If you are a smoker, then consider quitting and lastly, drink alcoholic beverages moderately.

The Benefits of Eating a Balanced Meal

Opting for a balanced diet to maintain a healthy weight is important in order to achieve weight loss since you are still supplying your body the right amount of vitamins and minerals it needs to function properly. When combined with consistent exercise, it is inevitable that you will lose weight without risking any health problems.

Maintaining a balanced diet with the aim of losing weight is beneficial as compared to products that promise a quick and easy way to weight loss. First, it lessens the risk of your developing cardiovascular diseases like heart diseases and diabetes. It can also aid you in controlling these conditions if ever you are suffering from one. This healthy regimen also promotes regular metabolism and a healthy digestive system, which will enable you to lose bad fats and absorb the good ones.

Aside from that, the choice of eating a balanced diet will definitely boost your confidence knowing that you will achieve your desired weight in the healthiest way possible.

How to Start Right

Starting out can be quite a challenge but it should be easy. Always remember the basics of eating more whole-carbohydrates by avoiding foods like chocolates, ice creams, chips, sodas, cookies, cakes and many others. These types of foods contain high amounts of sugar, cholesterol, salt and other unwanted substances.

These foods are also called 'empty calories' since they do not provide nutrients other than calories. Choose to drink fresh fruit juice instead of sodas, as they add approximately 500 calories more to your diet.

With that in mind, plan your meal correctly by adding more of the good kinds of food. You can have a high-fiber cereal with low-fat milk at breakfast, and then lunch would be a grilled turkey sandwich over whole wheat bread and a vegetable salad. Dinner can be baked fish and vegetables.

These are just a few of the simple dishes you can make and they are even easier to prepare. Just keep in mind that every meal should contain a variety of foods, such as fruits, lean proteins, vegetables and high-fiber carbohydrates.

CHAPTER 6- THE PRINCIPLES OF WEIGHT LOSS

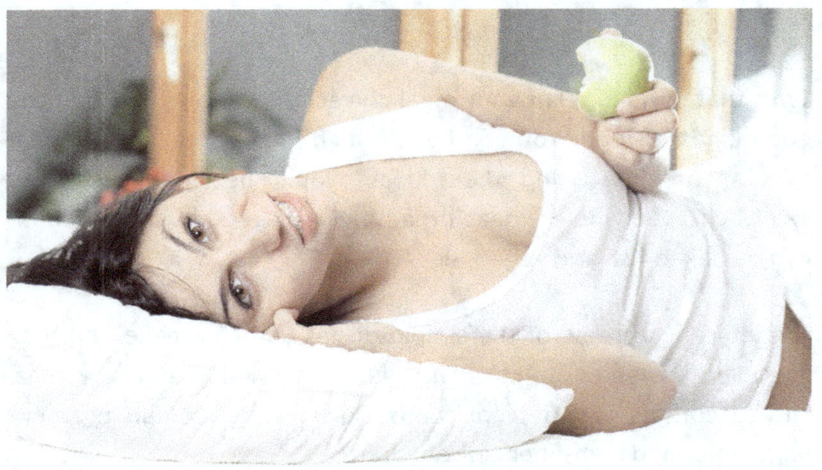

- **The Blood Type Diet**

A lot of people now understand the importance of having a healthy body. This is why there is a surge in the health and fitness industry. A lot more people are now going to the gym to try different forms of exercise to get in shape.

People are also trying different kinds of diets, from Atkins to Paleo to South Beach to Weight Watchers. All of these are effective, though some more than others. But did you know that there's a diet that is designed for your blood type? If you have tried almost all of the famous diet trends available and have not seen a lot of results, then this might be the perfect one for you.

This diet was designed by Doctor Peter D'Amado and is called The Blood Group Diet. This new diet is gaining more popularity because a lot of the big names in Hollywood say it's the reason for their amazing bodies. Actors like Courtney Cox and Cheryl Cole swear by it.

It is believed that each blood group reacts differently to each food. So if you follow the diet designed for you, the chances of losing weight will be higher because your body will absorb food more efficiently.

Let's look at the diet closely. If you have Blood Type O, which is the most common blood type in humans, then the diet should be similar to Paleo where it is encouraged to eat more like "hunter-gatherer" style. This means eating food that was available to our ancestors before agriculture growth and advancement in technology happened. High protein and low in carbohydrates is the way to go.

Along with this diet, blood type O people should also do a lot of high intensity cardio like running to complement the diet.

Blood Type A diet is almost the opposite of the diet suggested to Blood Type O. Meaning, their bodies are much more accepting to the more "modern" food. A vegan diet is encouraged, so this means lots of vegetables and carbohydrates like rice, pasta and cereals. However, meat and dairy products such as milk, cheese or butter should be avoided. Meat should be taken in very little quantity.

Blood type A diet is best done with slow and relaxing exercise such as yoga or Pilates.

Blood Type AB can be defined as the most lenient diet. This rare blood type works well with almost every food but with moderation. They have a good immune system, which means they can handle dairy, meat and carbs well. However, vegetables are the most encouraged food to eat. The rest should be eaten in little portions.

When it comes to exercises, Blood type AB should combine both calming and high intensity workouts.

Blood Type B has the least restrictions. Vegetables, fruits, meat, dairy, seafood, and rice - these can all be taken as long as it's part of a balanced diet and not taken in big quantities. The only foods to avoid are processed foods such as the ones that can be bought in a can (luncheon meat, hotdog, ham etc.)

Any activity that involves exercising the brain such as tennis, golf, and hiking is the best form of exercise for this blood type.

- **Real Carbohydrates Exist**

The first thing you need to do is to identify your carbohydrate intake. All of us know that carbohydrates are the main source of energy as carbs are readily converted to glucose, the main substance that is used for energy production. All the excess carbohydrates are turned into fat when they aren't used as energy. Now, what you need to remember is that you need to consume 'real carbohydrates' by choosing foods that are not processed. Replace the processed carbohydrates with natural ones like vegetables and fruits in every meal. Momentarily avoid other carbohydrates like chips, breads, pasta, fast food meals and others.

- **Choose High-Biological Proteins**

High-biological proteins are what you can think of as complete proteins. They are called such because they contain complete amino acids to provide efficient functions in terms of repairing body tissues and supplying proteins to every muscle in your body.

Amino acids work like a team: when one is missing, they cannot function well. So it is good to invest in high-biological proteins by eating natural and grass-fed meats and produce. This includes turkey, beef, chicken, lamb, pork and other animal proteins.

• Healthy Fats are for Real

If you think that fats are the only culprits of weight gain, you are definitely wrong. Your body also needs fats in order to function well as these substances contribute to temperature control, metabolism regulation and lubrication of vein and arteries. So, have a moderate intake of healthy fats, including avocadoes, coconut oil, olive oil, nuts, olives, seeds and butter. Just remember to consume about 2-3 teaspoons of these fats at every meal.

These are the three easy steps that you can always remember for you to have a significant weight loss. Start on these rules and you are off to a good start. It is good to remember that metabolism is as complex as our brain, so the notion of calorie counting does not really apply to all.

The basis of a healthy weight should come from consuming the right amount and kinds of food or to simply put it: the right balance of food. So start your meal right today by investing more on real carbohydrates, high-biological proteins and healthy fats.

• There are Right Kinds of Proteins

Proteins are essential to help tissues repair themselves and supply a leaner body structure. There are so many uses of proteins you may never know. In fact, they can also be used as energy when the carbohydrate sources are empty. Aside from that, they strengthen your immune system and give you skin that is smooth in texture. It has anti-aging benefits, enhances memory and so much more. This is why proteins are pretty valuable and should be saved for their functions instead of using them as energy.

Choosing the right kind of protein is essential to give you the advantage of having a lean body mass without the risk of sore muscles. The advice below is from an expert trainer, Taoist master Tommy Kirchhoff. He studied the popular martial arts Sheng Long Fu and is the Grandmaster of Victor Sheng Long Fu. He is a versatile fitness expert and is credited for contributing effective advice to fitness enthusiasts.

Not all have known this fact: proteins are made to function equally as compared to carbohydrates and fats.

So people are so wrong when they just invest in eating chicken alone. All proteins are a definite cure for intense training and they should be eaten in the most absorbable form.

Why?

This is because muscles need an immediate source of protein to supply their needs, especially during a heavy workout. With that, you need to opt for protein powders, as they give the quickest and most absorbable type of proteins to work and repair your body tissues. In order to find out which powdered proteins are best for you, just visit your personal trainer or sports nutritionist. You can also visit a sports house in your area or GNC stores.

Now, if you don't just have the right budget to buy these powdered proteins, which can be expensive by the way, you can opt for egg whites. The only thing that you should remember is this: you have to eat them raw and fresh.

Lisa Wright
Yes, you can get the most amino acids in raw fresh eggs as compared to cooking them. The reason for this is because as soon as you cook the egg, the structure of its proteins changes significantly, making it less absorbable. So manipulating an egg white, even if you shake, blend or stir them has effects that you may never know. In fact, your body may not even use the proteins completely.

Therefore, whenever you need the best proteins next to the powdered ones, get fresh eggs, separate the yolks (since they contain too much fat and cholesterol) and swallow them up.

Chapter 7- How Meal Timing Works

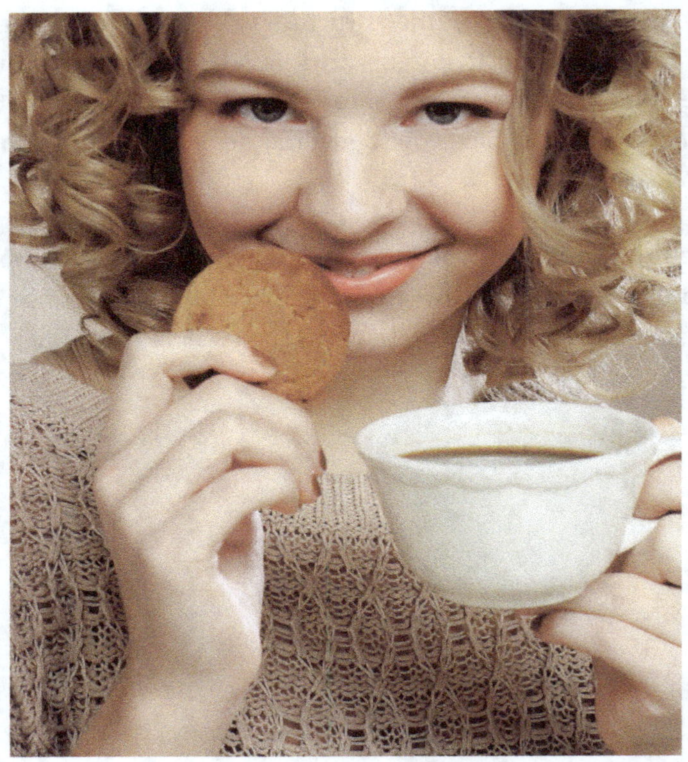

Meal timing is an essential part of a balanced diet. When we want to be on the top of our shapely figure, the right kind, amount and timing is important to balance your calories throughout the day. With that, there is no need to restrict yourself from eating lesser foods or depriving your body with the needed ingredients it should use for a day's work.

Our metabolism is different like our identity. Every individual has a different health and lifestyle profile which explains why it is hard to follow a single diet program.

A diet plan may be effective for you, but not for your friend. Even the intensity and duration of exercise may not be suitable for your friend as compared to yours. So to better understand what is actually happening inside your body, here is a basic explanation.

Breakfast Time:

- The body has fasted from sleep so there is no food intake for 8-12 hours.

- With this occurrence, the energy reserves (in the form of glycogen) are definitely low.

- This is where our muscles are in a state called mild catabolic, since the energy reserves are used for energy while there is no food intake for 8-12 hours.

- The fat stores are being used up as energy. Thus, it is being burned and mobilized.

Your metabolic goal at this time is to replenish the glycogen stores that were used from the fasting hours. You also need to stop your muscles from catabolism so that you will not acquire a state of muscle wasting. Along with that, you also need to support the continuous metabolism of fat.

To do that, you need to have a combination of high quality proteins that are absorbable enough to quickly replenish your muscles from fasting, like eggs and lean meats. You can also mix simple with complex carbohydrates to quickly replenish energy and at the same time, gradually release some of it as you go along your daily routine.

Fat is also important, so make sure to consume essential fatty acids. With that, you can eat walnuts, seeds and avocadoes. You can also make use of little amount of oil like canola oil or flax seed oil.

AM Snack

- The level of your glucose is already gradually balancing out

- The feeling of hunger is increased

Your metabolic goal: give your muscles the strength they need by consuming proteins and enough carbohydrates. It is good to further balance out your glucose level and at the same time, replenish protein stores.

To do that: You need to mix proteins and carbohydrates just enough to attain your metabolic goal. Consider foods with low-glycemic index and you can drink protein shakes, whey proteins from milk and fresh egg whites.

Lunch Time

- The morning snack that you have eaten is burned as energy and you may need more for a full day's work.

Your metabolic goal is to provide your muscles with sufficient calories with carbohydrates and proteins. Lunch can be your largest meal as compared to breakfast and dinner since you will work more after.

To do this, simply mix high-protein meat products like beef or chicken, then opt for high-fiber and low-glycemic carbohydrates. It is also good to invest in essential fatty acids.

PM Snack

- The levels of the glucose in your body are now deteriorating.

- With a few hours of mild fasting, your muscle is in a metabolic state again.

At this time, your metabolic goal is to gradually level your glucose up and stop the muscles from being catabolized.

To do this: Simply choose a snack that is enough to keep you replenished until dinner. Eat proteins that are slowly absorbed like cooked eggs. As for the carbohydrates, choose the ones that are low in sugar but are dense in calories.

Dinner Time

- Your muscles are anabolic as they prepare for another 8-12 hours of fasting during a sleep. This is up until about 12 in the morning.

Your metabolic goals should support your muscles while they are in an anabolic stage so the catabolic state will not impose any health problems in the long run.

With that, you need to eat types of foods that are low in calories but rich in protein. Choose proteins that are slowly absorbed like beef, pork and chicken. Invest in high-fiber carbohydrates and essential fatty acids.

Why You Should Eat the Right Kinds of Food

By now you should fully understand that healthy eating is not synonymous at all to dieting – and especially where dangerous fad diets are concerned. Eating the right food may be a struggle at the start, but it's a challenge that's guaranteed to promise numerous health benefits once healthy eating becomes a regular part of your life.

A Balanced Intake of Vitamins, Minerals, and Other Nutrients

By knowing which foods to eat more of and which ones to eat in moderation, you will be able to benefit from a balanced intake of vitamins, minerals, and essential nutrients. This may come as a surprise to you, but too much of any particular vitamin can actually be detrimental to your health.

Vitamin D toxicity, for instance, can lead to excess content of calcium in your body, which could be bad for your bones and heart. On the other hand, vitamin deficiencies are – as you know – just as bad. Hypocobalaminemia or Vitamin B12 deficiency can inflict long-term damage on nerve tissues if the disorder is not addressed and left untreated.

Higher Energy Levels

A lot of people have a hard time understanding the importance of energy because it's something you can't actually see. Even so, energy is something that will make a difference in how you feel especially as you advance in years. Higher energy levels allow you to be more physically active – especially compared to peers who haven't yet appreciated the benefits of healthy eating. You get to enjoy a better overall quality of life as well as spend a more productive time not just at work but when you spend time with your loved ones as well.

Stress Reduction or Elimination

People may not directly die of stress, but you can be sure that stress is one of the leading contributing causes to diseases that do kill. Stress doesn't just affect your health. It can also affect your career and personal relationships. Even the way you interact with your family may be negatively affected if you let stress get the better of you.

Thankfully, healthy eating is one of the best ways to combat stress. It puts you in a better mood and makes you less vulnerable to anxiety and depression.

Lower Blood Pressure

Hypertension is the other name for high blood pressure and is a symptom for many different types of chronic diseases. Most of those diseases affect your heart and may have life-threatening consequences. Maintenance for hypertension can be quite expensive and surgery for critical cases is even more cost-prohibitive. You can avoid all such headaches in the future, however, if you simply opt to do what's right now by eating healthy.

Diabetes

Some people still mistakenly assume that diabetes is something you can only suffer from when you're young. Others erroneously believe it's only hereditary. However, diabetes is a disease you can incur anytime and even if you do not like eating sweets a lot. There are other ways for your body's glucose levels to reach abnormal rates, but you can combat them effectively just by eating healthy.

How to Get Back Your Pre-Pregnancy Glory
Aside from those mentioned above, eating right can also help lower your risk for various types of cancer and heart diseases. As you can see, healthy eating is the first and best step you can take to enjoying a long, healthy and fulfilling life.

CHAPTER 8- GETTING RID OF A MOTHER'S NIGHTMARE – BELLY FAT!

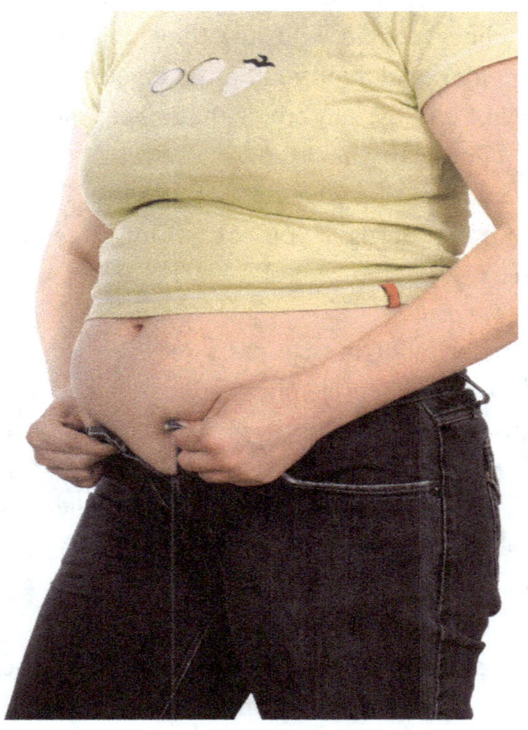

Usually, belly fat is subcutaneous fat, which is underneath the skin. If you have problems with abdominal fat, it may also be visceral fat. This is also known as organ fat that is packed between your internal organs. This is also known as the "pot belly" or the "beer belly." It is associated with type 2 diabetes, cardiovascular disease, and colorectal cancer.

In recent studies, scientists have come to realize that it isn't really how much a person weighs—it's their amount of body fat that truly indicates obesity. Throughout the 1980's and 90's imaging techniques were developed that helped improve the understanding of exactly how many health risks can be associated with the accumulation of body fat. These include tomography and magnetic resonance which help divide masses of tissue in the abdominal region.

For women, belly fat is more common after menopause. Sometimes, those people who just think this goes hand-in-hand with getting older, and don't realize the danger it can cause. While women feel like it is just something that makes them go up a size in their jeans, it does carry health risks. Like fat in any other area, it is determined by balancing your calories you take in with the energy you burn. In other words, if you eat too much and burn too little, you'll have excess fat.

As you get older, your muscle mass reduces. Your fat, however, increases. When your muscle mass reduces, it also reduces the rate your body uses calories. This can make it even more difficult for people to maintain a weight that is healthy as they age. Sometimes, you can have an increase of belly fat as you age without even gaining weight. In women, this can be due to a reduced level of estrogen.

Research has shown that estrogen seems to influence where the fat is distributed in a woman's body. Regardless of a weight shown as normal on the BMI measurement charts, women with a large waistline have been known to carry the risk of premature death and often dye earlier of cardiovascular disease. Most women hate to even have an inch or so too much belly fat. How do you know, however, if the belly fat you carry is a health risk? Just measure it. Use a tape measure and place it around your bare stomach. You want it to be snug, but not cut into the skin.

 For women, if your measurement is over 35 inches, you'll be at a greater risk for health problems. For men, the measurement of concern is around 40 inches. People who are plagued with belly fat often exercise and participate in healthy activities, yet they still retain that unwanted fat. It seems like the fat is immune to exercise. So how do you get rid of it? What is the magic combination that says "poof" to that extra poundage? It depends on your sex, age, and the amount of pounds you want to lose, but there are many tips to help you reduce that unwanted belly fat.

How to Reduce Belly Fat

Fortunately, belly fat can be eliminated or reduced by the same means that other fat can. It just takes the right combination of diet and exercise. There are, however, other factors that can hinder weight loss and cause you to retain belly fat. Below are some tips that can help you reduce that belly fat and have those abs you've always dreamed of:

1. Avoid stress

Research has found that our bodies produce hormones in response to stress. One of these is cortisol. It will cause your body to look for high-calorie food because it thinks it used a lot of energy handling something that was stressful. It's kind of like tricking your body into thinking it's had a big workout, when in fact, it's done nothing but become anxious and upset. Years ago, eating that type of high-calorie food was fine when you were stressed, because you used more energy every day working in the fields or on farms. Our ancestors remained thin during stressful times because of their hard work. Now, many of us live more sedentary lives. We simply can't burn that type of fat intake any longer. When you're under a large amount of chronic stress, it tells your body to keep on making cortisol. It becomes a vicious cycle.

Gaining weight makes you even more stressed, so you produce more cortisol and eat more fattening foods. You can reduce stress by doing several things. You can get more sleep. The average adult should get at least seven hours of sleep a night. You should keep things that are stressful away from the area you use for sleeping. Don't do work in bed if you can help it. That area should be for relaxation and rest instead of work. Simply work at leaving your worries outside the bedroom door. You should also set aside some time to relax each day. By closing your eyes, breathing deeply, and forgetting your worries for a brief period, even if it's only 15 minutes a day, you can help reduce stress. Exercise will also help by giving you an outlet for the stress. Keeping your blood sugar level will also help.

2. Tell friends/family that you're dieting

By telling others that you're dieting, you have them to help keep you in check. Of course, you'll hear things like, "You're dieting aren't you" or "Are you supposed to be eating that," but it will help you stick to your diet. You'll also hear things like, "How much have you lost" or "You're looking so good." Those things can be very encouraging. Once you've made the proclamation that you're dieting, you'll feel like you have to prove you can do it, so you're more apt to stick with it and achieve success.

3. Diet with a friend

Having a "buddy" system when you diet is a great way to lose weight. You have someone to help keep you in check, but you also have someone you can eat out with that you won't have to explain you're dieting to or someone that will be eating fattening foods in front of you. You can help and encourage each other along the way. You can celebrate each success you make as well as the success of your friends.

4. Heat your skillet when you fry

If you take the time to heat your skillet before you add the oil, the oil gets hot quicker and less oil will be absorbed by your food. If you put oil in a cold skillet, and add the meats or vegetables, oil will soak into the food. If it soaks into the food, where does it go? It goes right into your body and adds belly fat.

5. Use oats to stuff meat recipes

Use oats that are in the same amount of other things you fill with such as crackers or bread crumbs. Not only are oats better for you, because they have high fiber content, they taste the same, and can help you reduce your cholesterol.

6. Don't drown your food

You may or may not be old enough to remember Timer from the science portion of School House Rock watched in your Saturday morning cartoons. If you do, then you know he had a slogan: Don't drown your food in catsup or mayo or goo. It's no fun to eat what you can't even see, so don't drown your food! How many times have you seen someone prepare a nice, healthy salad only to pile on so much fattening dressing that it's no longer healthy? People will also pile on so much gravy that a lean piece of roast beef or turkey becomes unhealthy. Topping with meat natural juices instead or using extra virgin olive oil that is seasoned on salads will keep your food healthy and won't sacrifice the taste.

7. Keep frozen bananas on hand

Frozen bananas are great for making smoothies that are healthy and nutritious. They're sweet, so they eliminate the need for sugary ingredients. Frozen, they have the cold state for good thick smoothies and won't go bad quickly like they can if they're unfrozen.

8. Eat chocolate

Yes, you read correctly. So often, people ignore their cravings for chocolate because they feel it is "bad" for them. Dark chocolate, however, is lower in fat and very high in antioxidants, so eating it will both satisfy your cravings and give you a healthy snack. You can also shave dark chocolate into dishes like barbecue sauce or chili. It gives it a good flavor boost, and will help you prevent heart disease as well as keep your cholesterol at a good level. If you want a good night-time snack, take two tablespoons of dark chocolate and melt it in the microwave. Stir it with 4 ounces of vanilla yogurt and top it with about a tablespoon of almond slivers.

9. Purchase nuts that are in shells

If you have to spend time shelling the nuts, you'll spend less time eating big handfuls of them. Nuts in and of themselves can be healthy, especially pistachios, almonds and walnuts. If, however, you eat too many, they become like any other food you overeat and will cause you to gain weight.

10.   Boil your peanuts

If you boil peanuts for a few hours, they will have approximately four times the amount of antioxidants they have prepared any other way. Boiled peanuts are a popular snack already in Asia, China, Australia, and the southern portion of the US. If you haven't tried them, the next time you want peanuts, give them a try.

11.   Serve yourself water as an appetizer

Water is filling, cleansing, and keeps you properly hydrated. If you drink two glasses of water before each meal, you will fill up quicker and eat less.

12.   Add spice to your life

Research has found that people that were overweight will become slimmer if they eat meals that contain Chile peppers. They contain capsaicin. It's what makes them hot, and it helps the liver clear insulin from your bloodstream after you eat. Since insulin is the hormone that tells your body to store the fat, clearing it from the body can reduce belly fat.

13.   Avoid emotional eating

Sometimes people use food as a comfort. When you're hurt or upset, you turn to food to make you feel better. When you feel like eating just to eat and you know you're not hungry, substitute it with something else like going on a bike. If you must eat something, make it fresh fruits or vegetables.

ABOUT THE AUTHOR

Lisa Wright was a customer representative prior to her decision to turn her life around. She was overweight, eating donuts and drinking coffee throughout her shift to keep her awake. One day, her fiancé left her for another lady and was told that the reason he left was because she was too fat and ugly. This became the starting point towards a new life for her.

Lisa quit her job and studied to become a nutritionist and weight expert.

Today, she has the body she thought would never come to reality. She is in a happy relationship, and will finally walk down the aisle in a couple months' time.